All about the ketogenic diet
low in carbohydrates and rich in fats and proteins

Josh Motley

Introduction

The ketogenic diet also known as KETO DIET is a low carbohydrate diet that promises fast weight loss. The diet is based on a biochemical principle that regulates the functioning of our body: ketosis.

It is a drastic diet that must be observed and dictated only by specialized doctors. It is not a DO-IT-YOURSELF DIET because it modifies the processes of our organism. The diet is usually carried out for 21 days and a break period follows. Let's find out all about the keto diet, how it works, if it works and what are the contraindications.

What Is The Ketogenic Diet

This diet regime involves the drastic reduction of carbohydrates and the increase of proteins and fats.

This diet is usually used to lose weight, but we highlight that it is not a DIY diet that anyone can follow, it is a difficult diet to follow and must be followed by a specialist for it to work.

Ketosis

Ketogenic diet means in fact diet that produces ketone body.

The ketogenic diet is based on the drastic reduction of carbohydrates in the diet: but why? Carbohydrates are the energy source of cells to carry out any activity. If this energy is lacking, the body needs to find a substitute: with this diet it will be pushed to use fats as an energy source.

This process is called ketosis and leads to the formation of molecules called ketone bodies: ketosis is reached after a couple of days of restrictive diet with only 20-50 grams of carbohydrates consumed per day.

In order to perform all daily activities, our body metabolizes glycides, such as carbohydrates and sugar, which are found in the blood. If we suddenly deprive the body of these two elements, it will look for them in its own stocks present in the body in the form of fats.

Ketosis is then induced, the mechanism that prompts the body to burn its fat stores because it can no longer find carbohydrates and sugar.
Reaching ketosis and keeping it unaltered without causing damage is not easy and must be followed by a doctor.

Are we in ketosis? the first symptoms

After a couple of days ketosis should begin.
To understand that the body has entered into the state of ketosis you can perform a urine test with special strips or blood test using blood ketone meters or breathing by measuring the amount of ketones in the breath.
There are also some clear signs that may reveal to be in ketosis:
exhaustion
dry mouth and feeling of thirst
increased diuresis
acetonic breath or sweat due to the presence of acetone
reduced appetite

Various low carb diets

The ketogenic diet is mainly used to eliminate extra kilos: it only affects the fat mass and can achieve good results in a short time.
The keto diet has different methods that can be distinguished in :

hyperproteic ketogenic or Atkins diet;

normoproteic ketogenic or VLCKD diet used in cases of obesity

ketogenic normo-hypoproteic which is used not to lose weight but for the treatment of drug-resistant epilepsy

Keto

Ketogenic diet: how to reach ketosis

The ketogenic diet is a nutritional scheme that can be summarized as follows
low in calories
low percentage and absolute content of carbohydrates (low carb diet)
high percentage content of proteins
high percentage content of lipids
In order for the keto diet to work we must first induce ketosis: how?
The first step is to eliminate from the daily diet sources of carbohydrates, such as bread, pasta, potatoes and sugar products, but also dairy products, legumes, fruits and vegetables of orange and red color.
Only meat, eggs and fish are allowed in the ketogenic diet. Food supplements based on vitamins and Omega 3 can be added.
It is fundamental to drink a lot of water, at least two liters a day.
The classic food pyramid is completely overturned! Many proteins, few cereals and tubers.

Only by respecting the dietary regime imposed by the dietician can you reach ketosis: you can never deviate because it would be enough, for example, a candy to bring the body back to the previous balance and stop consuming fat to produce energy.

Ketogenic diet: what to eat

The ketogenic diet is a low-calorie diet, low carb, zero sugar, high content of proteins and lipids.
What do we eat during our initial three weeks on the diet?
A guideline of the proper ketogenic diet includes an energy breakdown of:
10% from carbohydrates
15-25% from protein
70% or more from fats
It is recommended to include supplements in the diet as well, in order to make up for the lack of minerals, omega 3 and vitamins.
Let's see now what to eat in quantity, what to eat less and what to give up.

What to eat in quantity

In large quantities you can eat all proteins of animal origin such as
meat, eggs and fish.
cheese
fats and oils for seasoning

vegetables such as: salad, broccoli, zucchini, spinach, cardoon, cauliflower, fennel, squash blossoms, radicchio, celery, green peppers, radishes, turnip greens, ribs.
What to eat in moderate quantity

You can eat but in limited quantities and recommended by your doctor:

vegetables such as: tomatoes, pumpkin, artichokes, green beans, eggplants, red and yellow peppers, asparagus, leeks and onions dried fruit, but to be consumed in small quantities.
fresh fruit only three times a week.

What not to eat

Avoid all cereals and cereal products such as
bread
breadsticks
crackers
sweets
pasta
Also to be avoided are: legumes, potatoes, fruit, sweet drinks, alcohol and foods that may include hidden sugars such as fruit juices, which contain 90% of added sugars and only 10% of pulp.

Beware also of sugars contained in candies, chewing gum, medications, supplements... just the accidental intake of sugars and ketosis stops: the body would go back to functioning as before and the effort made until then would be wasted.
An example diet for a week
Before starting such a diet, a professional should be contacted. It can be a very dangerous diet for our physique if not carried out under strict medical control.
With this diet regimen it is estimated the loss of 3 kilos per week.

A ketogenic diet is usually composed as follows

breakfast: two hard-boiled eggs with a side of sautéed vegetables or a slice of toast with cheese and avocado
lunch: a turkey burger with a side of cheese and avocado or salad with turkey, hard-boiled eggs, arugula, avocado, gorgonzola and croutons (30 grams)
snack: bananas, pineapple, apples, persimmons and mangoes in moderation or cheese
dinner: pork chops with a side of sautéed green beans or grilled salmon with a side of spinach

Ketogenic diet and physical activity

To accelerate and improve the process implemented with a low-calorie diet, it is always advisable to continue with an adequate physical activity. Even physical exercise must be recommended by a professional in order to achieve good results without weighing on a body that is already undergoing major changes.

It is generally recommended to train 3 times a week for at least 30-40 minutes: long walks at a steady pace, jogging in the open air, yoga or swimming practices are sufficient.

It should not be forgotten that doing sports during a period of high fatigue, such as it can be the beginning of a diet, helps because it frees the mind and reduces stress.

Contraindications of keto diet

There are conflicting opinions about the well-being that exercise can offer during a period of ketoacidosis. In fact, it is thought that sport can increase the weight of the ketogenic diet, which is however a metabolic forcing that already weighs on the body, even the youngest.

Be careful because intense physical exercise increases the energy requirements of glucose favoring the production and accumulation of ketone bodies.

Before engaging in sports activities, ask your dietician for advice first.

Ketogenic diet: Who can do it?

Being a rather stressful diet for the organism, it cannot be carried out for long periods of time and above all it is not suitable for everyone.

Who can follow a Keto diet? those who suffer from:

severe obesity;

mild obesity but complicated by type II diabetes, hypertension, dyslipidemia, metabolic syndrome, arthropathy

non-alcoholic hepatic steatosis

Who cannot follow the diet

The ketogenic diet cannot be recommended for those who

are pregnant or lactating

suffer from psychiatric and behavioral disorders

have type I diabetes

have had a myocardial infarction

suffer from liver and kidney failure

has alcohol and drug abuse

post-diet

Once the diet period recommended by the dietician is over, a couple of days of normal diet with the introduction of carbohydrates will be enough and ketosis will end quickly. The body quickly returns to function as before.

Usually for long-term maintenance carbohydrates are slowly reintroduced and alternate periods of ketosis with periods of non-ketosis.

Why it didn't work

Those trying the diet for the first time may not see results. Reaching ketosis is not immediate and it is not easy especially the first time.

Therefore, nutritional ketosis, the process that really burns fat and weight, is not always achieved.

What are the reasons for non-ketosis?

you still eat too much

you eat too little

you eat too much protein: keto is a moderate diet that aims at 20-25% of calories coming from proteins

you eat too many carbohydrates: you should consume 20-50 grams of net carbohydrates per day, not more

intolerance or allergy to some food. Sometimes food intolerances cause inflammation which in turn can lead to weight gain. While food allergies are serious things and we notice them almost immediately, food intolerances can be more insidious. Some of the most common food allergies include dairy, eggs, peanuts, tree nuts, wheat, soy, fish and shellfish.

Another reason the body does not go into ketosis may be resistance to leptin. Leptin is the hormone that alerts the brain that the body is satisfied with the meal, that you are full. It is therefore essential to be able to regulate the consumption of daily meals especially is essential during a low-calorie diet. If this hormone is not functioning well it is also difficult to communicate the sense of satiety to the brain and this can be the cause of unmotivated appetite.

Leptin resistance is often caused by irregular sleep, stress, overeating and caloric restriction. In the case of leptin resistance it may be necessary to wait before seeing even the slightest benefit related to the ketogenic diet, even eight weeks to start seeing results.

Ketogenic diet: contraindications

The ketogenic diet used against obesity almost always leads to excellent results in the loss of fat mass. It must be followed by a specialist, it is not a do-it-yourself diet.

It is in fact known that this diet has different contraindications. What are the main contraindications of the Keto diet:

ketosis is considered a toxic condition for the body: the disposal of ketone bodies above the normal amount can in fact cause a fatigue of the kidneys;

maintaining the state of ketosis during the whole treatment is really difficult. It is enough to ingest a single forbidden food to compromise the state of ketosis and push the body to draw energy from sugars

initially the weight loss is evident but it is very difficult to maintain the weight achieved. There is a high risk of regaining all the lost pounds when introducing carbohydrates again. Post dieting is really complex and foods must be reintroduced into one's diet gradually. The maintenance period must be followed by a dietician doctor

ketosis may cause discomfort such as nausea, reduced appetite, dizziness, headache, fatigue, difficulty in breathing, constipation, excessive diuresis, sweat and acetoxy breath

is a diet that cannot be followed for long periods of time because it is not completely balanced and would damage the health;

it may cause: hypoglycemia, hypercholesterolemia and hypotension. Therefore, the patient must be controlled by a doctor.

remember: avoid do-it-yourself diets. if you intend to follow any diet, not only the keto diet, always consult your doctor and a nutritionist, so that they can provide you with tailored advice.

KETO CRESCENT DOGS

Perfect for game day, Keto Crescent Dogs are family-friendly, incredibly delicious and loaded with fat. Think of them as indoor, keto-style pigs. Create a delicious dough with mozzarella cheese, cream cheese, eggs and almond flour. Cut the dough into strips and wrap each strip around one of your beef hot dogs. Place them in the oven for 20-30 minutes and take them out just before opening the kickoff for a fantastic lunch.

REAL TEXAS CHILI

If you're looking forward to some spicy chili, this mouthwatering keto-adapted version of True Texas Chili will have you begging for more. The dish pairs 100% grass-fed beef with onions, red and green peppers, and beef broth, and includes rich spices like cilantro, paprika, and chili powder. With a mixture of curly cauliflower and Oaxaca cheese, this chili takes the taste to a whole new level. The best part about this dish, is that Ketoned Bodies will deliver it right to your door.

FRIED CABBAGE WITH CRISPY BACON

The quick prep and cooking time make Fried Cabbage with Crispy Bacon a fan favorite among all the keto lunch ideas we've collected. Simply cut the cabbage and bacon into small pieces, fry the bacon in a skillet, and then add the cabbage, butter, and seasoning, and voila! Healthy, quick and full of fat and flavor, this dish is sure to satisfy.

BEEF FA-KETO DISH

This meal is another Mexican dish that is simply loaded with flavor. Made with 100% grass-fed tri-tip beef, this meal also includes seasoned cauliflower rice, sautéed onions and peppers, and plenty of Mexican spices. With pico consisting of tomatoes, serrano peppers, cilantro, cumin, lime juice, and black pepper, the flavors of this dish jump out at you.

EASY KETO SWEDISH MEATBALLS

If you like those delicious meatballs at IKEA, then you'll love these. These Easy Keto Swedish Meatballs recipe is low-carb, gluten-free, and overflowing with fat. These meatballs are perfect for the whole family and are pretty easy to make at home. Mix ground pork and meatball

breadcrumbs, use finely grated zucchini to add texture to the meatballs. Roll them up and cook them on the stove in butter. Next, pour over a mixture of chicken broth, mustard and cream and simmer for 5 to 10 minutes. These meatballs go well with cauliflower rice.

Craving a sandwich, but don't want all the carbs that come with bread? Try a Keto BLT with Oopsie Bread . To make the Oopsie Bread, start by separating the egg yolks from the egg whites. Beat the egg whites with salt until very stiff. Add the cream cheese to the egg yolks. If you want, you can also add the psyllium seed husk and baking powder. Once the two mixtures are respectively mixed and ready, fold the egg whites into the yolk mixture. Bake 8 small Oopsies at a time. To make your BLT, fry up some bacon, cut up some heirloom tomatoes, fresh lettuce and basil. Spread a little mayo on the Oopsie bread, put the sandwich together and enjoy!

PULLED PORK WITH MANGO SAUCE

The pork is slow-cooked for more than 12 hours and the mango salsa consists of mango, red peppers, cilantro, lime, garlic and avocado oil. The meat and sauce sit on a bed of red and green cabbage mixed with bacon, and topped with Oaxaca cheese. If you're craving a delicious and vibrant tropical variation of pulled pork, this dish is definitely worth trying.

CAULIFLOWER CASSEROLE TWICE BAKED KETO

Cheese is the name of the game when it comes to this dish. This Twice Baked Cauliflower Casserole Keto is loaded with an array of decadent and fatty ingredients, including full-fat cream cheese, sour cream, Parmesan and cheddar cheese. Pair these wonderful ingredients with bacon and you'll go crazy. Incorporate garlic, green onions and whipping cream to make the dish even more heavenly.

KETO TUNA SALAD WITH HARD-BOILED EGGS

Fresh and delicious, this Keto Tuna Salad with Boiled Eggs is a great number to add to your arsenal of keto lunch ideas. Celery, shallots, tuna, lemon, mayonnaise and mustard are mixed with the tuna to make a zingy salad. Boiled eggs seasoned with pepper are also included on romaine lettuce. The whole thing is then drizzled with olive oil. It all makes for a quick, light and tasty keto meal.

STEAMED MUSSELS WITH PIRI PIRI

If you're looking for a dish with a Latin American flavor, this Steamed Mussels with Piri Piri recipe features a chimichurri-style sauce made with red onions, parsley, red wine vinegar, garlic, jalapeño, crushed red pepper and olive oil. Steam the mussels in white wine and water and top with Piri Piri sauce for a unique high-fat, low-carb meal.

CASHEWS AND BROCCOLI

Take your typical Chinese takeout to new keto friendly heights with 100% grass-fed beef, seasoned with sea salt, cilantro, paprika, turmeric and garlic. Along with broccoli florets and beef, this Cashew and Broccoli also includes bacon, cashew sauce, sherry vinegar, almonds and coconut. Someone from Ketoned Bodies is happy to deliver this dish to you as part of one of our easy keto meal plans.

LOW-CARB KETCHUP STEAK WITH BLUE CHEESE ONION CREAM SAUCE

A nice juicy steak is the perfect lunch option that will keep you full all day long. This low carb steak with blue cheese onion cream sauce will have your mouth watering throughout the cooking process. Cook some Ribeyes in butter until they are medium rare. Next, sauté some onions in a generous amount of butter. Reduce them to a simmer and pour in some heavy cream. Melt in some blue cheese. At serving time, pour a generous portion of the sauce over the steak.

Keto Dinner

Lemon and Sage Creamed Chicken

Given its low fat content and high protein levels, chicken isn't always the best choice for a keto diet. But with a little tweaking, you can make up the difference and create a succulent ketopollo dish that will keep the ketones gushing. Lemon and sage creamed chicken (from Mark's Daily Apple) is one such meal. Bone-in chicken thighs roasted in a sauce of cream, cinnamon, garlic, lemon and sage make a delicious dish that really delivers in the health-fat department. And, at only ~30 minutes prep time (plus 45 minutes cooking time), you won't have to rearrange your schedule to accommodate this keto-chicken recipe.

Fried salmon with asparagus

Some easy keto dinner recipes are easier than others, and this one in particular may be the easiest of them all. This quick keto fried salmon with asparagus recipe from Diet Doctor has just three ingredients: salmon, asparagus, and butter, all fried together in one pan. Of course, that doesn't mean you can't

can build on the basic recipe; feel free to mix in other low-carb vegetables, and serve it all with garlic butter. The meal only takes about 10 minutes from start to finish (including cooking time), so keep the ingredients on hand and cook them when you need keto dinner ideas in a pinch.

Easy Stuffed Peppers

There are two sides to keeping carbs down: one is to avoid carbs in the first place, and the other is to increase your fiber intake. In simpler terms, fiber is something akin to an anti-carb, subtracting from total carbs. So, low carb, high fiber meals are certainly some of the best keto recipes you can get. With that in mind, check out this recipe for easy stuffed peppers from Keto Connect . Cut some poblano peppers lengthwise, fill them with some keto-friendly ingredients, and bake them in the oven for ~20 minutes, and you'll have an easy keto dinner recipe perfect for bringing down your net-carb count.

Keto Pizza Meatballs and Mushrooms

This is one of our favorites here at Keto Bodies - so much so that we now offer it as one of our products. This recipe was originally adapted from Maria Emmerich's 30-Day Keto Cleanse cookbook, available on Amazon in spiral bound, paperback or Kindle download. This Keto Pizza Meatballs and Mushrooms dish is flavorful and filling. Ingredients include 100% pasture-raised ground pork, mushrooms, onions, bell peppers, avocado oil, pasteurized eggs, red pepper flakes and organic garlic. And with 57 grams of fat, 21 grams of protein and only 7 grams of carbs, this meal is a keto dicter's dream come true.

Salmon with Pistachio Pesto

Wild salmon is perfect for the ketogenic diet - it's packed with vitamins and minerals, high in healthy fats, and moderately high in protein. And (as the best keto recipes tend to be) it's almost completely carb-free. This particular dish, Salmon with Pesto of
pistachio from Mark's Daily Apple The dairy-free, pistachio-rich pesto offers a hint of lemon and garlic, and is thick enough
to spread. You can add some salmon to the pan and then add the sauce, and you have a new take on traditional seafood. Alternatively, if salmon isn't your thing, you can use this pesto sauce on a variety of other meats and vegetables.

Deconstructed Pork Eggs

Another of Maria Emmerich's recipes that we've adapted here at Ketone Bodies , the Deconstructed Pork Egg-Roll is a worthy addition to our meal delivery menu. It's tasty. It's fun. And everything about egg rolls reworked in a way that's friendly. The all-organic egg roll filling contains pork, coconut oil, garlic, ginger, coconut oil, sea salt, chili flakes and a variety of delicious spices. It comes complete with a fresh kale blend and is keto's answer to those Chinese food cravings.

Best Keto Brownies

If the idea of a keto dinner has you stumped, wait until you try to find some keto desserts! The good news is that chocolate,
when done right, is a keto-friendly solution to the carb-shaped hole in your diet. That's why these Best Keto Brownies (from
Keto Connect) are so perfect. No sugar. Lots of butter. Three eggs. Unsweetened cocoa. What more could you want? With only 3 net carbs, you'll wonder how in the world this keto dessert tastes so good. And while brownies aren't dinner idea (per se), there's nothing stopping you from

incorporating these easy, delicious, sweet and fudgy brownies into the

Keto Chicken BLT Salad

A good salad is a great way to go for easy keto dinner recipes, and this keto chicken BLT salad (from Diet Doctor) is as good as it gets. A classic BLT sandwich may not be totally keto friendly, but replace the bread with some leafy greens and add some chicken thigh and garlic mayo, and you're in keto town. The prep time for this sandwich is around 15 minutes, so as long as you have the ingredients ready and have access to a pan (for the bacon and chicken), you don't have to plan this meal too far in advance. Just be sure to take precautions when handling raw chicken, or substitute in some pre-cooked roast chicken.

Boneless pork chop and zucchini spears

A juicy pork chop paired with some low carb veggies is enough to make almost any keto dieter's mouth water. That's why Ketoned Bodies has included this boneless pork chop and Zucchini Spears dish as part of our keto delivery menu. The pork chop is 100% organic pasture-raised boneless and comes with a spice rub consisting of sea salt, paprika, cilantro, onion powder, turmeric, garlic and black powder. Perfectly grilled, with a flavorful char and a succulent center, this pork chop meal includes zucchini spears and crushed cauliflower as a side dish so you can enjoy some good fiber along with your fats and protein.

Meatloaf and red pepper glaze on the sides

Bread may be a keto no-no, but you can still enjoy a loaf - meatloaf ...that is. And when it comes to Mama Meatloaf and sides the meal with Ketoned Bodies' red pepper glaze, have fun on is exactly what you'll be doing. Combining 100% beef grass-fed with green peppers, eggs, onions, heavy cream and more, and topped with a delicious red pepper glaze, this meatloaf is a great way to celebrate dinner while hitting your macros. The broccoli and crushed cauliflower sides bring in some extra vitamins and fiber and help round out the whole experience.

Wonton Soup

If you think about it, the only thing keeping traditional wonton soups from fitting into the keto diet are the wonton wrappers; get rid of them, and you're in business. So that's exactly what this recipe from Mark's Daily Apple does. This delicious wonton soup recipe hollows out the carb-rich wraps and has you roll the ground pork filling right into little meatballs. Cook them in the recipe's chicken broth stock and serve them all together with raw baby spinach or baby bok choy. Feel free to add chopped green onions and chili oil if you want a little more kick.

Chicken Saltimbocca

For many people, Italian food and the ketogenic diet simply don't mix. But3
what these people need to remember is that Italian food is more than just pasta with carbs. Take this easy Saltimbocca Chicken recipe (from Keto Connect) for example. A combination of chicken, ham and spinach, this recipe offers Italian flavors without the Italian carbs. The end result is a mouthwatering, delicious meal that sticks you with only 1.3 grams of net carbs per serving. And, if the ingredients listed are too expensive, or if you want to add your own personal touch, this recipe is easy to adapt to any taste.

Chicken Jambalaya Sausage and Andouille

Rice is pretty high in carbs, so before you can enjoy traditional rice meals on the keto diet, you need to find something to replace it. Cauliflower rice makes this possible, and is the perfect ingredient to complement the Ketoned Bodies Chicken and Andouille Sausage Jambalaya. This "dirty rice" dish will have you cleaning up your plate. Blending pork sausage, chicken thighs, and chicken liver with a variety of spices and low carb vegetables, this cajun treat will have your taste buds fluttering on your back, but won't break your body out of ketosis.

Keto Asian Noodle Bowl

Just like pasta and rice, Asian noodles are some of the first things a keto dieter will have to learn to give up before becoming fully fat adapted. Miracle noodles change all that, offering an Asian-noodle substitute with zero net carbs. And now, with this recipe from Keto Connect You can use these noodles to create a Keto Asian Noodle Bowl with all the flavor and satisfaction of traditional ramen. Incorporating chicken, eggs, mushrooms, scallions, pink salt, and a delicious marinade, this noodle bowl will make you rethink Asian noodles. However, it does require a little more prep time than some of the other easy recipes on this list, so be sure to take that into account when planning your meals.

Keto Scramble with Sausage

Eggs are a dieter's best friend - they're high in fat, contain moderate protein, and are essentially carb-free. But what makes them such a boon is that they're also easy to adapt to many different dishes.

Scramble with sausage from Ketoned Bodies is one such meal. Scrambled eggs mixed with sausage, cheese, red peppers, and more make a flavorful and filling meal perfect for breakfast or dinner. And, if you decide to create your own variation, you can easily add other low carb vegetables and high fat meats. All you need are some organic eggs, a pan and some of your other favorite keto ingredients.

Snak Keto

when you want to lose weight, usually the first foods to be eliminated are carbohydrates. in fact, a balanced diet should never be devoid of any nutrient, because they are all essential for our health and well-being. but we know that abusing carbohydrates leads to a rise in the glycemic index that certainly does not help you lose weight, so it is important to know how to combine foods for a healthy diet.

to dishes rich in whole carbohydrates, it is necessary to combine low carb snacks in the mid-morning and in the afternoon, to break the hunger and avoid binge eating during meals.

snacks, which, as mentioned, should never be missing from a healthy and balanced diet, are good, quick and give us an immediate sense of satiety. you can focus on snacks without carbohydrates: an excellent source of protein and fiber, vitamins and minerals and, perhaps during the heat and the summer, also rich in water.

Good and bad carbohydrates: what they are and how to choose them

But which are those that have a low carbohydrate content and allow us to eat without getting fat?

Fresh fruit in season

Apples, bananas, strawberries, oranges, tangerines, peaches or apricots are perfect for your low carb snack. Remember to prefer the raw version with the peel to store all the available nutrients.

Centrifuged drinks

To these natural drinks made from fruits and vegetables, you can add half a glass of semi-skimmed milk for a higher protein intake.

Dried Fruits

Walnuts, almonds, hazelnuts and pistachios as well as being excellent snacks (please do not exceed 30-35 grams), are an excellent source of antioxidants, vitamins and minerals.

Yogurt

Natural, low-fat, with fresh fruit or pieces, or accompanied by 30 grams of cereals, yogurt is one of the best low carb snacks!

Vegetables

Vegetables are a good alternative to fruit, as they provide a good supply of fiber, vitamins and antioxidants with very few calories. Try mixing sweet veggies like carrots, squash, arugula, radicchio, radishes, beets, celery and cucumbers, add a pinch of ginger and you're done.

Wheat, oats, and rye can be a great low carb snack, but instead of buying pre-made bars at the grocery store, why not try making your own? It's super easy!

21 Days Plan

WHAT IS THE KETOGENIC DIET AND HOW DOES IT MAKE YOU LOSE WEIGHT IN 10 TO 21 DAYS

The ketogenic diet, also known as the 21-day diet, is a dietary regimen almost devoid of carbohydrates (intake less than 5%) that triggers the so-called ketosis. This is a particular metabolic state in which the body, not having carbohydrates available, is forced to burn fats for energy production. By doing so, weight loss is accelerated in a short time.

During a ketogenic diet it is necessary to drastically reduce the intake of carbohydrates, almost to the point of elimination (less than 5%); on the contrary, an abundant intake of fats is preferred. In the field of nutrition, this translates into some precise types of food.

THE KETOGENIC DIET: A SCIENTIFIC APPROACH

The ketogenic diet is a dietary regimen in which there is a drastic reduction of carbohydrates in favour of proteins and fats. This operation induces in the body the formation of acid substances called ketone bodies, such as beta-hydroxybutyrate, acetic acid and acetone. The production of ketone bodies occurs physiologically in conditions, for example, of fasting.

Normally the cells in fact need glucose for their regular functions, but if the supply of the latter is reduced to excessively low levels, they will begin to activate compensation mechanisms, with reduction of insulin and activation of catabolic processes.

After a couple of days of fasting, in fact, there is a depletion of glycogen stores with a consequent stimulus to gluconeogenesis and ketogenesis, which will lead to the formation of ketone bodies usable by the brain.

Therefore, the cells, in particular the nervous ones, will use these substances as a primary source of energy. This metabolic state is called "nutritional ketosis", and is considered a fairly safe state, since ketone bodies are produced in small concentrations without significant alterations in blood pH.

It differs greatly from ketoacidosis, a life-threatening condition in which ketone bodies are produced in extremely higher concentrations, altering blood pH and thus causing acidosis.

Typically ketosis is reached after a couple of days with a daily carbohydrate intake of about 20-50 grams, but these amounts may vary on an individual basis.

FOR WHOM THE KETOGENIC DIET IS INDICATED

Severe or complicated obesity (hypertension, type 2 diabetes, dyslipidemia, OSAS, metabolic syndrome, osteopathy or severe arthropathy)

Severe obesity with indication for bariatric surgery (in the pre-operative period)

Patients with indication for rapid weight loss due to severe comorbidities

Non-alcoholic fatty liver disease (NAFLD)
Drug-resistant epilepsy.

CONTRA-INDICATIONS OF KETOGENICS

Pregnancy and lactation
Positive history of mental and behavioral
disorders, alcohol and other substance abuse
Hepatic or renal failure
Type 1 diabetes
Porphyria, unstable angina, recent AMI.

EVIDENCE SUPPORTING THE KETOGENIC DIET

(by the Faculty of Pharmacy, University Federico
II of Naples)
Carbohydrates now represent about 55% of the
typical diet, but it is known that a high intake of
sugars is associated with an increase in the
prevalence of obesity and metabolic syndrome, as
well as an increased risk of developing diabetes
mellitus. Recent studies in the literature have
compared the long-term effects of dietary
interventions on weight loss, showing no strong
evidence to recommend low-fat diets. In fact,
reduced carbohydrate diets have been shown to
achieve significantly greater weight loss than the
former. In addition, individuals following a
ketogenic diet initially experience rapid weight
loss of up to 5 kg in 2 weeks or less, which is why
we often hear the term "10-day or 21-day diet".

This dietary regimen also has a diuretic effect, reducing the sense of hunger and it is interesting to note how it often determines a saving in the use of muscle protein mass for energy purposes.

Fish, preferably wild (anchovies, swordfish, squid, octopus, cuttlefish, sea bream, sea bass, shrimp, cod, salmon);
Quality meat (chicken, veal, turkey, rabbit, beef);
Eggs, prepared in any manner;
Green leafy vegetables and Vegetables (asparagus, mushrooms, cabbage, chicory, spinach, zucchini, fennel, cucumber, eggplant, artichokes);
Fatty cheeses and dairy products;
Cold cuts;
Liquids: still water, coffee and unsweetened herbal teas, broth;
Snacks: fennel, pure licorice, take dima10g as a snack (in this case dose from a single scoop)
Condiment: 30ml of oil daily, salt without exceeding, apple cider vinegar (but not white vinegar/balsamic vinegar).

There is also a group of foods to be consumed only in moderation:
Certain vegetables (tomatoes, peppers, garlic, onion, eggplant);
Certain fruits (mainly red fruits and lemon), to be consumed no more than 3 times a week;
Rye bread;
Dried fruits, nuts, almonds;
Some beverages such as tea and coffee.

On the other hand, there are several foods that cannot find any place in the ketogenic diet, so they should be avoided completely:
Bread, pizza, pasta, rice, corn, barley and all other products made from wheat flour or cereals;
Potatoes;
Legumes;
Sugar of any kind;
Foods containing added sugars and sugars (also avoid sugar-free candy);
Sugary drinks, fruit juices, beer, alcoholic beverages.

Here is a daily ketogenic diet menu to be followed with a protein supplement (such as dima10g). The cycle should last from 10 to 21 days.
Breakfast: 2 scoops of protein (dima) dissolved in 200ml of water (or in 200ml of skimmed zero fat milk or in white Greek yogurt) + bitter coffee (or bitter tea);
Lunch: 2 scoops of protein (dima) in water;
Snack: fennel or pure licorice or Dima 10g (one scoop);
Dinner: chicken thighs and artichokes (or sea bass and beets or two eggs and broccoli baresi or steak and green salad).

The following is an example of a food menu to be applied as a first reintegration for 15 days, that is, after finishing the first ketogenic cycle.

Breakfast: 200 ml of skimmed milk without sugar, or low-fat yogurt, or orange juice;

Mid-morning snack: 1 low-fat yogurt;

Lunch: 50/70g of spelt or brown rice with vegetables 1 portion of vegetables at will

Snack: 1 protein bar (such as Dimabar)

Dinner: 200/300g of white meat roasted eggplant or zucchini.

Here is an example of a day's food to be applied as a stabilization for 15 days, or after several ketogenic cycles completed and in anticipation of a longer stabilization before following others.

Breakfast: 200 ml of skimmed milk, or yogurt 200 g, orange juice;

Mid-morning snack: 200g of fruit;

Lunch: 100g bresaola 50g whole wheat bread 200g vegetables;

Snack: protein snack bar (Dimabar);

Dinner: 200/300g lean roasted meat 200/300g roasted mushrooms

Here is an example of a food day of 1300 kcal based on a ketogenic regime, recommended for 7 days after a stabilization phase and in anticipation of a resumption of the ketogenic cycle:

Breakfast: 1 pot of white Greek yogurt (125 g) + 50 g of ham with 1 slice of rye bread;

Mid-morning snack: dried fruit 30 g;

Lunch: fish or lean meat (200 g) with a side of vegetables (150 g) seasoned with EVO oil (15 g) + Whole wheat bread 30g

Snack: fennel or pure licorice or Dima 10g (one scoop);

Dinner: omelette of 2 eggs + vegetable side dish (150g) + EVO oil 15g + a small fruit.

We can simplify the ketogenic diet into 4 main phases:

carbohydrate deprivation

onset of ketosis

acceleration of weight loss and production of ketone bodies

elimination of ketone bodies through diuresis

In phase 1) the deprivation of carbohydrates is started by following the diet we have talked about.

The diet (also facilitated by the use of supplements, see below) will induce the organism to a state of ketosis in the first 3-4 days (phase 2). During this period the organism is stressed and may experience drops in energy, fatigue and exhaustion. If this occurs, it is advisable to remain under the control of your doctor and nutritionist of confidence, so that you can take advantage of an energy vitamin complex.

Phase 3) At this point comes the best part: the body is burning fats as a source of energy and in this way there is an acceleration of the slimming process, which involves critical points, such as the belly, thighs, arms and hips (phase 3). The output of ketosis is the production of ketone bodies, which must be biodegraded by the body.

In phase 4) we have the elimination of ketone bodies through urine. It is advisable from the beginning of the diet to use a specific draining supplement.

[HOW MUCH CAN YOU LOSE IN 10 DAYS]

The first tip with the ketogenic diet is not to look at the scale in the first 10 days. This is a method that tends to "deflate" hard-to-reach parts of the body, and this is regardless of weight. Also to answer the question we have patients who have lost as much as 7-10kg with the first 21 day ketogenic cycle. The subjective matebolism can vary the results, but we can conclude that with the ketogenic cycle you lose from 4kg to 10kg in about two weeks (10-21 days)

See testimonials and opinions of those who have followed the ketogenic cycle

WHEN IS KETOSIS REACHED?

Generally, ketosis is reached after 2-3 days with a daily amount of carbohydrates of about 20-50 grams. There is variability depending on the individual's metabolism.

[HOW CAN I TELL IF I'M IN KETOSIS?]

significant reduction in appetite;

dry mouth;

acetonic breath;

sense of fatigue (use a multivitamin to counterbalance).

[WHAT VEGETABLES CAN BE EATEN DURING THE KETOGENIC DIET?]

All green vegetables are allowed and can be eaten (except green beans), in the amounts provided. So asparagus, mushrooms, cabbage, chicory, spinach, zucchini, fennel, cucumber, eggplant, artichoke.

[HOW MANY POUNDS CAN YOU LOSE IN A WEEK AT MOST?]

If ketosis is induced properly, with a responsive metabolism, the body goes into ketosis after three days of carbohydrate deprivation. Therefore in the following 4-5 days it starts to burn fat as an energy source. When this circuit works properly we have verified an average loss of 2-4kg in the first week.

HOW MUCH CAN YOU LOSE IN ONE NIGHT?

Fast slimming, if approached in a rigorous and scientific way, allows you to lose weight in a week, in 10 days, in a month. Even reaching strategic areas of fat accumulation, such as the hips, belly, face, which are usually difficult to "sculpt". But slimming in one night does not fall into this category and is unlikely to bring benefits whatever you do. In particular, the ketogenic diet requires a cycle of at least 10-21 days to produce positive effects.

For more info on fast slimming consult the mainstay article of our blog that continues numerous resources, diets, methods and tips to lose weight in a short time: How to lose weight fast

Lightning Source UK Ltd.
Milton Keynes UK
UKHW021958030621
384904UK00002B/609